Mediterranean Amazing Recipes

Delicious Cooking Ideas for Your Daily Mediterranean Meals

Marta Jackson

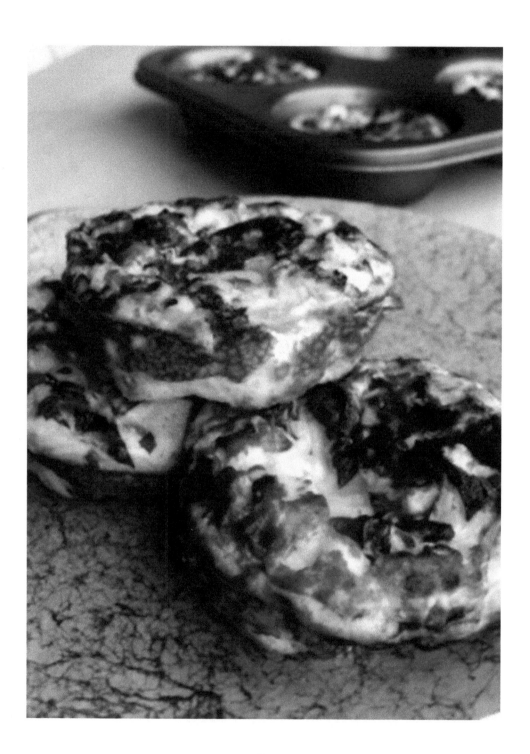

By reading this document, the reader agrees that under no circumstances is the author responsible for any losses, direct or indirect, which are incurred as a result of the use of information contained within this document, including, but not limited to, — errors, omissions, or inaccuracies.

Table of Contents

Mexican street corn

This corn is no ordinary corn, it is accompanied with chili powder, lime and mayonnaise for a better taste to suit the Mediterranean Sea diet taste. It works as a snack or an appetizer.

Ingredients

- ¼ teaspoon of kosher salt
- 2 ounces of finely grated Cotjia cheese
- ¼ cup of mayonnaise
- 2 tablespoons of finely chopped cilantro
- 1 ½ teaspoons of lime juice
- ½ teaspoon of chili powder
- Pinch of cayenne pepper
- 4 ears of grilled corn on the cob

Directions

- In a small bowl, combine the mayonnaise together with the lime juice, chili powder, cayenne, and salt. Stir to combined.
- In another separate bowl, mix together the cheese with the cilantro. Set both aside for later.

- Brush the mayonnaise mixture all over one ear of corn.
- Sprinkle the Cotjia mixture liberally all over, turning the corn as needed.
- Place the finished cob on a separate serving plate.
- Repeat this step for the remaining corn.
- Sprinkle a pinch of additional chili powder lightly over the corn.
- Serve and enjoy when still warm.

Best guacamole

Ingredients

- 3 tablespoons of lime juice
- ¼ cup of finely chopped fresh cilantro
- 1 teaspoon of kosher salt
- 1 small jalapeño, seeds and ribs removed
- ½ cup of finely chopped white onion
- 4 medium ripe avocados
- ¼ teaspoon of ground coriander

Directions

- Scoop the flesh of the avocados into a serving bowl.
- Then, mash up the avocado until smooth to your expectation.
- Next, add the onion together with the cilantro, coriander, jalapeño, lime juice, and salt. Stir until combine.
- Taste, and adjust the seasoning to your taste.
- Serve and enjoy.

Avocado pesto toast

Avocado is one of the few Mediterranean fruits blessed with the gift of nourishing the skin. As a result, this recipe featuring tomatoes and garlic for a flavor is adequate for your skin nourishment needs.

Ingredients

- Cooked eggs
- 2 large ripe avocados
- Freshly ground black pepper, red pepper flakes
- 2 medium cloves garlic
- 2 tablespoons of lemon juice
- Halved cherry tomatoes
- ¼ teaspoon of salt
- ¼ cup of pepitas
- ⅔ cup of packed fresh basil leaves
- 4 slices of organic bread

Directions

- Place the pepitas into a small skillet.
- Let cook over medium heat, stirring frequently until making little popping noises.

- Then, transfer to a bowl, let cool.
- Scoop avocado flesh into a bowl of a food processor.
- Place the garlic together with the lemon juice, and salt.
- Blend until smooth.
- Add the toasted pepitas with the basil leaves and pulse until the pepitas and basil are broken down.
- Taste, and adjust seasoning accordingly.
- Spread a generous amount of avocado pesto over each slice of toasted bread.
- Serve and enjoy.

Sweet potatoes and black bean tostadas

This is a complete vegetarian Mediterranean recipe with roasted sweet potatoes serve beautifully on a bed of crisp salad.

Ingredients

- Salt
- Small handful of fresh cilantro leaves, chopped
- Extra virgin olive oil
- 1 teaspoon of ground cumin
- 2 cans of black beans, rinsed and drained
- Hot sauce or salsa
- ½ cup of water
- 2 cloves garlic, pressed
- 2 ripe avocados, pitted and thinly sliced
- ½ teaspoon sea salt grinder
- 8 corn of tortillas
- 18 ounces of romaine lettuce, roughly chopped
- 1 ¾ pounds of sweet potatoes
- ⅔ cup of feta cheese crumbles
- ½ teaspoon chili powder
- ¾ cup of finely chopped red onion, divided

- 2 tablespoons of fresh lime juice

Directions

- Preheat the oven to 400°F.
- Line baking sheets with parchment paper.
- Place the sweet potatoes on baking sheets, drizzle with olive oil, and sprinkle with the chili powder and dash of salt. Toss to coat.
- Let bake for 35 minutes, or until the sweet potatoes are tender and caramelized.
- Warm olive oil over medium heat, until shimmering.
- Then, add the garlic and cumin, let cook briefly, while stirring constantly.
- Add drained beans, water and salt. Let simmer and cook for 10 minutes, stirring often.
- Remove from the heat and mash the beans, cover and set aside.
- On a baking sheet, brush both sides of each tortilla with oil.
- Arrange 4 tortillas in a single layer across each pan.

- Let bake for 12 minutes, turning until each tortilla is golden. Keep aside for later.
- In a medium serving dish, combine the chopped lettuce together with the feta, red onion, olive oil, and lime juice. Toss to combine.
- Divide the salad between 4 bowls.
- Serve and enjoy immediately.

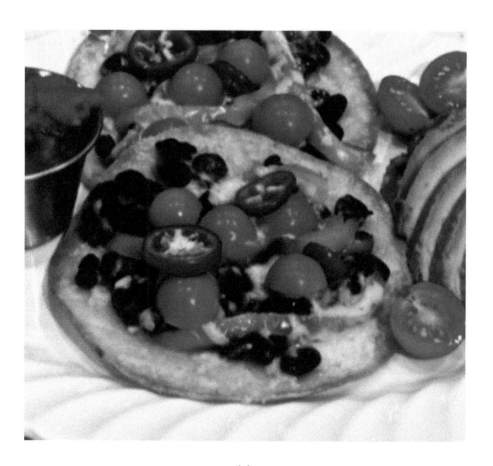

Kale, black bean, and avocado burrito bowl

Ingredients

- 3 cloves garlic, pressed
- ¼ teaspoon of salt
- 1 bunch of curly kale
- ¼ teaspoon of chili powder
- 2 tablespoons of olive oil
- ½ jalapeño, seeded and finely chopped
- ½ teaspoon of cumin
- Cherry tomatoes, sliced into thin rounds
- ¼ teaspoon of salt
- ¼ cup of lime juice
- 1 cup of brown rice, rinsed
- 1 avocado
- ½ cup of mild salsa Verde
- ¼ teaspoon of cayenne pepper
- ½ cup of fresh cilantro leaves
- Hot sauce
- 2 tablespoons of lime juice
- 2 cans of black beans, rinsed and drained

- 1 shallot, finely chopped

Directions

- Bring a big pot of water to a boil, lace in the brown rice and boil, uncovered, for 30 minutes.
- Drain any excess water, return to the pot. Let steam in the pot for 10 minutes, season with ¼ teaspoon salt and adjust accordingly.
- Whisk the lime juice together with the olive oil, chopped jalapeño, cumin, and salt.
- Toss the chopped kale with the lime marinade in a mixing bowl.
- Combine the avocado chunks, salsa Verde, cilantro, and lime juice in a food processer, blend well.
- Warm 1 tablespoon olive oil over medium-low heat.
- Sauté the shallot together with the garlic until fragrant.
- Add the beans with chili powder and cayenne pepper.

- Let cook until the beans are warmed through in 7 minutes.
- Serve and enjoy.

Sweet corn and black bean tacos

Beans are rich in protein; therefore, combining with variety of vegetables and fruits makes this recipe a perfect choice for Mediterranean Sea diet.

Ingredients

- 1 large avocado, sliced into thin strips
- Salt and black pepper
- 3 medium red radishes, thinly sliced into small strips
- ¼ cup of chopped cilantro
- 1 medium jalapeño pepper, seeded and minced
- 1 tablespoon of olive oil
- Pickled jalapeños, salsa Verde
- ¼ teaspoon of sea salt
- 2 ears of corn, shucked
- ⅔ cup of crumbled feta, to taste
- 1 medium lime, zested and juiced
- 2 cans of black beans, rinsed and drained
- 10 small round corn tortillas
- 1 tablespoon of olive oil
- 1 small yellow or white onion, chopped

- 1 tablespoon of ground cumin
- ⅓ cup of water

Directions

- Place the kernels in a medium-sized mixing bowl with jalapeño, olive oil, chopped cilantro, radishes, lime zest and juice, and sea salt. Mix well.
- Then, stir in crumbled feta, taste, and adjust.
- Warm the olive oil over medium heat.
- Add the onions with a sprinkle of salt, let cook 8 minutes, stirring occasionally.
- Add the cumin, let cook briefly while stirring.
- Pour in the beans and ⅓ cup water. Stir.
- Lower the heat, let simmer, for 5 minutes, covered.
- Smash half of the beans.
- Remove from heat, then, season with salt and pepper.
- Heat a cast iron over medium heat and warm each tortilla individually, flipping occasionally.
- Serve and enjoy.

Lemony broccoli, chickpea, and avocado pita sandwiches

Ingredients

- Pinch red pepper flakes
- 1 can of chickpeas, rinsed and drained
- 2 medium avocados
- 4 whole grain pita breads
- ⅓ cup of finely chopped red onion
- ⅓ cup of crumbled feta cheese
- ⅓ cup of oil-packed sun-dried tomatoes, rinsed and chopped
- ¼ cup of olive oil
- ¼ teaspoon of salt
- 2 tablespoons of lemon juice
- 1 ½ teaspoons of Dijon mustard
- 1 bunch of broccoli, florets removed and sliced thin
- 1 ½ teaspoons of honey
- 1 clove garlic, pressed or minced

Directions

- In a medium mixing bowl, combine broccoli, chickpea, sun-dried tomatoes, red onion, and feta cheese. Toss to combine.
- In a small mixing bowl, combine olive oil, lemon juice, Dijon mustard, honey, garlic, salt, and peppers. Whisk to emulsified.
- Taste, and adjust the seasoning accordingly.
- Pour the dressing over the broccoli chickpea salad, let toss to combine. Allow it to marinate.
- Scoop the avocado flesh into a bowl, mash until they are spreadable.
- Season with a pinch of salt.
- Warm pita bread in microwave and spread each slice with mashed avocado.
- Serve and enjoy.

Portobello mushroom and poblano pepper fajitas

Ingredients

- 2 tablespoons of fresh parsley
- ¼ cup of olive oil
- ½ lime, juiced
- 1 small jalapeño, finely chopped
- ½ teaspoon of ground cumin
- ¼ cup of lime juice
- Sea salt and black pepper
- 2 tablespoons of water
- ½ teaspoon of ground coriander
- 10 corn tortillas
- ¼ teaspoon of ground chili powder
- ⅓ cup of fresh cilantro
- 2 avocados
- Sea salt and black pepper
- 3 large Portobello mushrooms, rinsed and pat dry
- 1 medium purple onion
- 4 medium poblano peppers

- ⅔ cup of crumbled feta cheese

Directions

- Begin by tossing the slices of Portobello mushroom, poblano pepper, and onion into a large bowl.
- In a small bowl, whisk together olive oil, lime juice, jalapeno, cumin, coriander, chili powder, salt, and pepper to emulsify.
- Pour the marinade over the bowl of prepared veggies. Toss well.
- Let the veggies soak the marinate for 30 minutes.
- In a food processor, combine the avocados together with the cilantro, parsley, lime juice, and water. Blend, and season with sea salt and black pepper.
- Transfer to a small serving bowl.
- Heat a tablespoon of olive oil over medium heat.
- Add in the marinated vegetables once the olive oil is shimmering, let cook, stirring occasionally, until the peppers are tender.

- Remove from heat.
- Warm the tortillas individually in a lightly oiled pan over medium-low heat, flipping halfway through cooking.
- Stack the warmed tortillas on a plate and keep them warm under a tea towel.
- Serve and enjoy with tortillas and or avocado sauce.

Veggie breakfast sandwich

The vegetable breakfast sandwich recipe has versatile choice of toppings. It uses variety of vegetables and fruits mainly avocado.

Ingredients

- 2 teaspoons of mayonnaise
- Thinly sliced red onion
- ½ ripe avocado, mashed
- Salt and freshly ground black pepper
- 1 slice of ripe red tomato
- 1 large egg
- Small handful of arugula
- ½ teaspoon of water
- 1 teaspoon of butter or olive oil
- 2 small slices of cheddar
- 1 whole wheat muffin, sliced in half and toasted
- Several dashes of hot sauce

Directions

- Start by spreading the mayonnaise over the lower half of the toasted muffin.

- Then, spread the mashed avocado over the other half, and sprinkle it with a bit of salt and pepper.
- Heat a medium non-stick skillet over medium-high heat.
- In a bowl, scramble the egg with water and bit of salt and pepper.
- Add a pat of butter and swirl the pan to coat the bottom once the pan is hot.
- Pour in the scrambled egg and immediately swirl the egg in the bottom of the pan to make an even layer.
- Place the cheese in the center of the egg mixture, then, fold one side of the egg over the middle, then the opposite side over the middle.
- Place the cooked egg on the mayo-covered bun, topping with a slice of tomato.
- Add with several slices of red onion, a few dashes of hot sauce, and a little handful of arugula.
- Top with the remaining bun, avocado side down.

- Serve and enjoy.

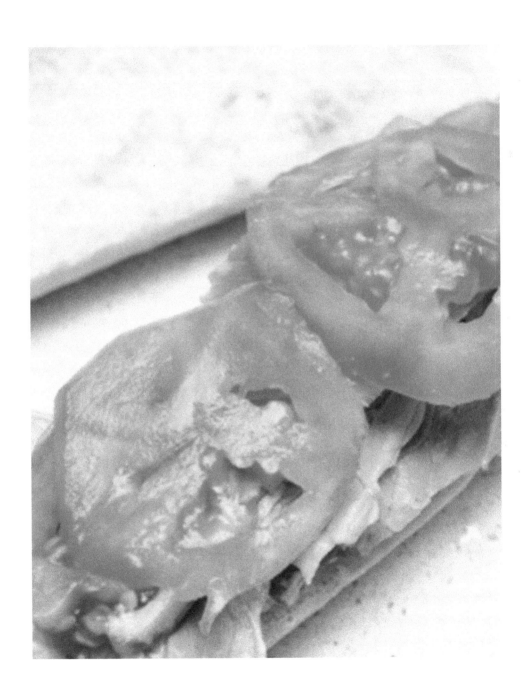

Sweet potato burrito smothered in avocado salsa Verde

Ingredients

- ½ teaspoon of cumin
- ¼ teaspoon of cayenne
- Sea salt and black pepper
- 6 whole wheat tortillas
- Sour cream
- 2 roasted red peppers
- Sea salt
- Chopped jalapeño
- ½ teaspoon of smoked hot paprika
- 1 ½ cups chopped romaine lettuce
- 2 cups cooked black beans
- 2 ripe avocados
- 2 medium sweet potatoes
- 1 cup mild salsa Verde
- 2 garlic cloves, roughly chopped
- 1 small red onion
- 2 tablespoons of extra-virgin olive oil
- 2 teaspoons of fresh jalapeño

- 1 lime, juiced
- ¼ cup of packed cilantro leaves

Directions

- Start by preheating the oven to 450°F.
- Toss the sweet potatoes together with the olive oil, smoked hot paprika, cumin, cayenne pepper, and salt and pepper.
- Place the sweet potatoes onto a large baking sheet lined with parchment paper.
- Let bake for about 45 minutes, flipping the sweet potato chunks halfway, until golden and caramelized.
- Combine the avocado flesh together with the salsa Verde, garlic, jalapeño, and lime juice in a blender. Blend.
- Add the cilantro and blend again.
- Taste, and adjust the seasoning accordingly.
- Place the tortillas on a baking sheet lined with parchment paper.
- In the middle of each tortilla, put down a couple strips of roasted red pepper, pour ⅓ cup

black beans down the center, topping with ⅓ cup of roasted sweet potato chunks.

- Let bake for 5 minutes on the middle rack, until the cheese is melted.
- Transfer each burrito to a plate, then smother in avocado sauce and sprinkle with ample romaine lettuce.
- Serve and enjoy

Simple Greek avocado sandwich

Ingredients

- 6 pitted Kalamata olives, thinly sliced
- ½ of an avocado
- 1 tablespoon of basil pesto
- Balsamic reduction
- Thinly sliced red onion
- Roasted red bell pepper
- Handful of spring mix
- 2 slices of soft whole wheat bread
- Cucumber, sliced into thin rounds

Directions

- Smash the avocado smooth enough for easy spreading.
- Spread avocado on one slice of bread.
- Spread a layer of pesto on the other slice of bread.
- Top the avocado bread with a single layer of roasted red bell pepper.
- Add a layer of cucumber slices, olives, red onion, and spring mix.

- Use a spoon to sprinkle some balsamic reduction over the lettuce.
- Place the pesto slice on top, pesto side down.
- Serve and enjoy.

Autumn couscous salad

Ingredients

- 1 ½ cups of apple juice
- 8 ounces of Israeli couscous
- ¼ cup of canola oil
- 1 tablespoon olive oil
- 1 tablespoon of parsley chopped
- ½ cup of dried currants
- 1 shallot diced
- 3 tablespoons of red wine vinegar
- kosher salt and pepper
- 1 fennel bulb diced
- 2 ½ cups of butternut squash peeled, seeded and diced
- 3 tablespoons of fresh sage chopped
- ¾ cup of dried cranberries

Directions

- Start by bringing water to boil in a medium size saucepan.
- Then, add couscous and bring back to a boil.

- Lower the heat, continue to cook for 8 minutes or until al dente.
- Drain excess water in a colander. Set aside to cool for later.
- Heat olive oil over medium high heat in a large sauté pan.
- Add the shallot let cook for 1 minute, stirring often.
- Add diced fennel, continue to cook for 5 more minutes.
- Add butternut squash together with the sage, cranberries, currants, and apple juice, let cook until butternut squash has softened.
- Season with kosher salt and pepper.
- Transfer the mixture to the bowl with the couscous, reserving some.
- In another separate small mixing bowl, mix the reserved apple juice together with the canola oil, red wine vinegar, and bit of salt and pepper.
- Add to the couscous with the parsley and stir.
- Serve and enjoy.

Garlic soup with sherry

The garlic soup with sherry draws its delicious taste from the smoky paprika and dash of dry sherry. It is purely vegetable with garlic as the main flavor with herbs.

Ingredients

- 4 eggs
- 6 cloves of garlic, peeled
- 6 cups of cubed French bread
- ¼ teaspoon of sweet pimento
- 4 tablespoons of extra virgin olive oil
- Salt to taste
- ¼ cup of minced parsley
- 6 cups of chicken broth
- 3 tablespoons of dry sherry

Directions

- Begin by heating the chicken stock in a pot.
- Sauté the garlic cloves on low heat, stirring until golden.
- Sauté the bread in the remaining olive oil until browned and crusty.

- Crush and add the garlic cloves to the broth.
- Add bread together with the paprika, sherry and salt.
- Heat the broth to a boil, lower the to medium.
- Crack each egg into a small bowl.
- Pour the eggs to rest in the soup.
- Cover the pot and poach the eggs until the whites are firm.
- Serve in bowls with an egg in each and garnish with parsley.
- Serve and enjoy.

Sautéed greens with onions and tomatoes

The sautéed greens with onions and tomatoes is a Mediterranean master of vegetables and greens. It blends in variety of kingly ingredients mainly garlic, leek, cayenne pepper, and paprika.

Ingredients

- 1 ¼ cups of snipped fresh dill
- 1 teaspoon of cayenne pepper
- 1 ¼ kg of fresh mixed tender greens.
- ¼ cup of extra virgin Greek olive oil
- 2 tablespoons of tomato paste
- 2 leeks washed well and finely chopped
- 2 garlic cloves minced
- 2 teaspoons of sweet paprika powder
- 1 ¼ cups of snipped fresh wild fennel leaves or mint leaves
- 2 large onions halved and sliced
- 1 cup of plum tomatoes peeled and finely chopped
- Salt and freshly ground pepper

Directions

- Blanch and drain the greens completely.
- Heat the olive oil in a large skillet, cook the onions with leek over medium heat, stirring, for 7 minutes.
- Add the garlic together with the tomato paste, cayenne, and paprika, stir for 3 minutes or so.
- Add the wilted greens with dill, wild fennel leaves, and tomatoes.
- Let simmer over low heat, for 20 minutes uncovered.
- Taste and adjust the seasoning with salt and cayenne.
- Pour a little fresh olive oil over the greens once they are cooked.
- Serve and enjoy.

Barbunya pilaki; beans cooked with vegetables

Ingredients

- 3 tablespoons of olive oil
- 2 cups of water
- 2 cups of dried borlotti beans
- 1 lemon, cut in wedges
- 1 medium to large onion, finely chopped
- Salt and freshly ground black pepper
- 2 medium carrots, quartered and chopped in small cubes,
- 1 can of good quality canned chopped tomatoes
- Handful of flat leaf parsley, finely chopped
- 2 teaspoons of sugar

Directions

- Start by soaking the dried borlotti beans prior to the day of cooking.
- Drain the beans, rinse and transfer and boil in a pot partially covered for 35 minutes.

- Drain any excess water, rinse the cooked beans under cold water, keep aside for later.
- Heat olive oil in the pot, then stir in the onions, sauté for 3 minutes.
- Add the carrots, and sauté for 2 more minutes.
- Stir in the canned tomatoes with sugar.
- Season with salt and freshly ground black pepper. Combine.
- Add the beans to the pot and give it a good mix. Then pour in the water.
- Bring the pot to the boil.
- Lower the heat, then cover the pan partially.
- Let simmer for 35 minutes, until the beans are cooked
- Serve and enjoy at room temperature.

Braised okra recipe

Ingredients

- 500g of fresh okra
- 2 tablespoons of red wine vinegar
- ½ a cup of olive oil
- 1 onion finely chopped
- 500g of fresh pureed tomatoes
- A handful of chopped, fresh, flat leaf parsley
- Salt and pepper

Directions

- Prepare the okra.
- Sprinkle with red wine vinegar, let rest for 1 hour in a bowl.
- Drain and rinse with cold water.
- Heat olive oil in a heavy saucepan.
- Then, sauté onion over a low heat until to soften.
- Add the okra and toss in the olive oil together with the onion mixture for 5 minutes.
- Add the tomatoes with parsley, season to taste.
- Bring the mixture to a boil on high heat.

- Let simmer for 30 minutes on a low heat.
- Once the okra is tender serve and enjoy with crusty bread.

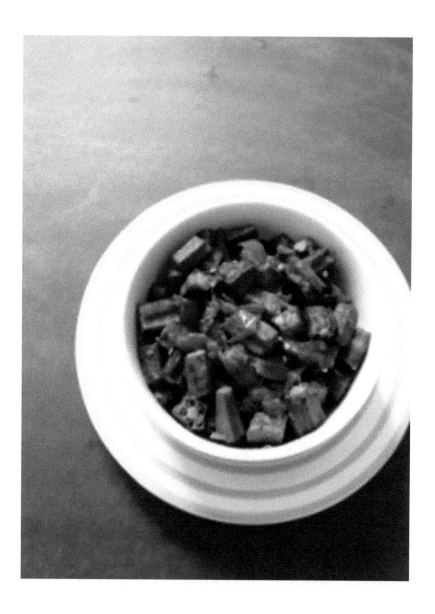

Louvi black eyed peas

Ingredients

- 1 teaspoon of flour
- 250g of black eyed beans
- 3 tablespoons of parsley, finely chopped
- 3 tablespoons of parsley, finely chopped
- 1 bunch of silver beet or chard
- 1/3 cup of lemon juice
- 1 medium onion, finely chopped
- Freshly ground black pepper
- 1 tablespoon of dill, finely chopped
- 1 spring onion, finely chopped
- 1 clove garlic, finely chopped
- ¼ cup olive oil
- 1 tablespoon of dill or fennel fronds
- Salt
- 4 cups of water

Directions

- Place black eyed beans in a pot and boil for 15 minutes.
- Drain any excess water.

- Then, sauté the onion with garlic in olive oil, then add silver beet and stir.
- Add the black eyed peas, let season with salt and pepper.
- Add water to cover all ingredients.
- Bring to boil, lower the heat, then simmer until the beans are soft.
- Toward the end add the parsley and dill and mix.
- Dissolve the flour in the lemon juice.
- Add to the mixture. Cook for a few more minutes.
- Serve and enjoy.

Greek style zucchini blossoms

Ingredients

- 2/3 cup of chopped parsley
- 1 cup olive oil
- Salt and pepper
- 1 cup of chopped onion
- 1 cup of chopped chives
- 3 tablespoons of chopped fresh mint leaves
- 3 cloves, minced garlic
- 3 cups of yogurt
- 25 zucchini blossoms
- 1 cup of grated zucchini
- 1 cup of bulgur
- 2/3 cup of raisins
- 1 teaspoon of chili pepper
- 1 ½ cups of water
- ½ cup of pine nuts

Directions

- Heat half of the olive oil over medium heat and sauté the onion, chives, and garlic for 5 minutes, or until soft.

- Add the zucchini together with the bulgur, raisins, chili pepper, and 1 cup water.
- Lower the heat, then let simmer for 10 minutes.
- Add the pine nuts, mint, and dill to the stuffing when the heat is off.
- Season with salt, stir, and adjust accordingly.
- Stuff each blossom using a spoon.
- Fold the top over and place on their sides in an earthenware casserole.
- Pour the remaining olive oil and ½ cup water.
- Cover the dish and place in the oven.
- Let bake for I hour or so.
- Serve and enjoy hot or cold, according to your liking.

Mushroom, chorizo, and haloumi tacos

This recipe has unforgettable combination of a true and healthy Mediterranean Sea diet vegetables. It is quite wonderful with homemade tortillas.

Ingredients

- 8 tortillas, medium-sized and warmed in a pan
- 500g of button mushrooms
- 1 tablespoon of chilies, finely chopped
- 3 tablespoons of olive oil
- 1 teaspoon of salt
- 125g of chorizo sausage
- 200g of haloumi cheese
- 1 teaspoon of black pepper
- 1 tablespoon of coriander, finely chopped
- 1 pinch of oregano, dried

Directions

- Combine the mushrooms together with the olive oil, salt, pepper, and oregano in a bowl.
- Place on baking tray and cook in an oven heated to 400°F for 35 minutes.
- Remove, let cool briefly.

- Preheat a little oil, cook the chorizo on a medium high heat briefly until crispy. Set aside.
- In the same pan, fry the halloumi for 2 minutes on each side until, browned.
- Cut the haloumi into small even slices.
- Combine the mushrooms, chorizo and haloumi in a separate bowl.
- Pace 3 tablespoons of the mushroom mixture into a warmed tortilla.
- Garnish with fresh chilies and coriander.
- Serve and enjoy.

Chicory and beans

Ingredients

- Olive oil
- 3 medium heads of chicory
- Salt
- 3 cloves of garlic
- 1 small can of cannellini
- 1 pepperoncino

Directions

- Boil the chicory in salted water for 10 minutes, or until fully tender.
- Drain any water, reserving some for later.
- Squeeze dry and chop the chicory roughly.
- In a large sauté pan, lightly brown the garlic in abundant olive oil, adding the pepperoncino or red pepper flakes for a few moments at the end.
- Remove both garlic and pepperoncino.
- Add the chopped chicory to the seasoned oil and let it simmer for 5 minutes.
- Then add the canned beans with a ladleful of the reserved cooking water. Mix well.

- Let the mixture simmer again briefly.
- Taste, and adjust the seasoning.
- Serve and enjoy with a drizzle of olive oil.

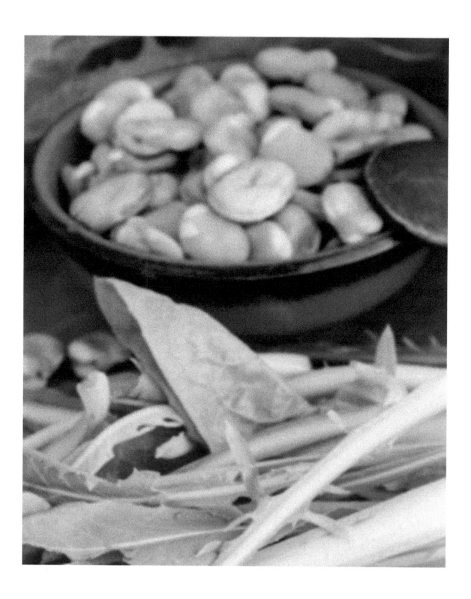

Smoked salmon with poached eggs on the toast

Ingredients

- 2 eggs, poached
- Splash of Kikkoman soy sauce
- 2 slices of bread toasted
- 1 tablespoon of thinly sliced scallions
- ½ large avocado smashed
- ¼ teaspoon of freshly squeezed lemon juice
- Pinch of kosher salt and cracked black pepper
- Microgreens
- 3.5 oz. of smoked salmon

Directions

- Smash the avocado in a small mixing bowl.
- Add the lemon juice and a pinch of salt, mix well and keep.
- Poach the eggs, when they are sitting in the ice bath, toast the bread.
- Spread the avocado on both slices of toasted bread, then add the smoked salmon to each slice.

- Transfer the poached eggs to their respective toasts.
- Hit with a splash of Kikkoman soy sauce and some cracked pepper.
- Place slice of tomato on each toast.
- Serve and enjoy.

Vegetarian potato skin egg boats

Ingredients

- 1 cup of shredded cheddar cheese
- 4 russet potatoes
- Fresh or dried chives
- 2 tablespoons of olive oil
- 8 large eggs
- Coarse kosher salt and freshly ground black pepper
- 2 teaspoons of smoked paprika

Directions

- Begin by preheating your oven ready to 450°F.
- Place potatoes on a baking sheet and pierce each one a few times with a fork.
- Let bake for 60 minutes.
- Remove, and let cool enough to handle.
- Raise the heat to 475°F.
- Slice each potato in half lengthwise.
- Scoop out the flesh, leaving ¼ inch of potato around the edge.

- Brush both sides lightly with olive oil and bake cut side down for 16 minutes, flipping halfway through.
- Lower the heat to 375°F.
- Season the inside of the potato skins with salt, pepper, and smoked paprika.
- Divide cheese evenly amongst the potatoes, then crack one egg into each.
- Sprinkle with chopped chives.
- Return the potatoes to the oven, let bake until the yolks jiggle slightly in 17 minutes or so.
- Serve and enjoy.

Baked eggs skillet with avocado and spicy tomatoes

Ingredients

- Vege-Sal and fresh-ground black pepper
- 1 10 oz. can of tomatoes
- 1 ripe avocado, sliced lengthwise
- 4 eggs

Directions

- Preheat your oven to 400F.
- Break eggs into individual ramekins and let the eggs come to room temperature.
- Brush a medium sized ovenproof pan with oil.
- Add the tomatoes, start to simmer over medium heat.
- Turn off the heat once all the liquid has evaporated from the tomatoes
- Arrange the avocado slices like spokes of a wheel in the pan.
- Place each egg between two avocado slices, spacing them evenly.

- Season with salt and fresh-ground black pepper.
- Place the skillet into the pre-heated oven, let bake until whites are completely set and the yolks are done in 10 - 13 minutes.
- Serve and enjoy hot.

Chard, mozzarella, and feta egg bake

Ingredients

- 8 eggs, beaten
- ¼ cup of sliced green onions
- 8 oz. of Swiss chard leaves, sliced into thick ribbons
- 1 teaspoon of Spike Seasoning
- 2 teaspoon of olive oil
- 3/4 cup of Mozzarella cheese
- Salt and fresh ground black pepper
- ½ cup of crumbled Feta cheese

Directions

- Preheat your oven to 375°F.
- Spray a glass casserole dish with olive oil.
- Cut stems off the chard leaves and discard stems.
- Stack up the leaves in a pile and cut the chard into ribbons.
- Then, heat olive oil in a heavy non-stick frying pan.

- Add the chard ribbons all at once, let cook while stirring until the chard has wilted and slightly softened in 3 minutes.
- Layer the wilted chard together with Mozzarella cheese, and Feta cheese in the bottom of the casserole dish sprinkled with green onions.
- Beat the eggs with the spike seasoning, salt, and pepper.
- Pour over the chard.
- Let bake until the egg bake is set and starting to lightly brown within 40 minutes.
- Serve and enjoy with a dollop of sour cream.

Bacon spinach and sweet potato frittata

Ingredients

- 1 cup of shredded cheddar cheese
- ¼ lb. of bacon
- large handful of baby spinach
- ½ cup of milk
- 1 large sweet potato peeled and cut into disks
- Kosher salt to taste
- 1 med onion diced
- 6 eggs

Directions

- Cook the bacon in a large oven-proof skillet over high heat.
- When ready, remove the bacon to a paper towel lined plate, keep aside.
- Lower the heat to medium, then add the onions to the same skillet with the bacon drippings.
- Let the onions cook for 2 minutes, then add the potato slices.
- Sprinkle with salt, let cook for 3 minutes on each side.

- Whisk the eggs together with the milk.
- Add salt and pepper, set aside for later.
- Preheat your oven to broiler low.
- When the potatoes are slightly browned and soft, sprinkle them with baby spinach.
- Pour the egg mixture on top and then sprinkle with the cooked bacon.
- Top with shredded cheese, let continue to cook over medium low heat, until the eggs start to set in 10 minutes.
- After 8 minutes, lift the edges of the eggs to allow the liquid to run down underneath.
- Transfer the pan to the oven.
- Broil until lightly browned.
- Slice, serve and enjoy.

Spinach and mozzarella egg bake

Ingredients

- 8 eggs, beaten
- 5 oz. of organic fresh spinach
- salt and fresh ground black pepper
- 2 teaspoon of olive oil
- 1 teaspoon of spike seasoning
- 1 ½ cups of grated mozzarella cheese
- 1/3 cup of thinly sliced green onions

Directions

- Preheat your oven to 375°F.
- Spray a glass casserole dish with olive oil.
- Then, heat the olive oil in a large frying pan.
- Add spinach all at once, and stir just until the spinach is wilted.
- Transfer spinach to the casserole dish, spreading it around to cover the dish bottom.
- Layer the grated cheese and sliced onions on top of the spinach.
- Beat the eggs with spike seasoning, and salt and fresh ground pepper

- Pour the egg mixture over the spinach combination
- Then, let bake for 35 minutes or until the mixture is completely set.
- Let cool for 5 minutes.
- Serve and enjoy when hot.

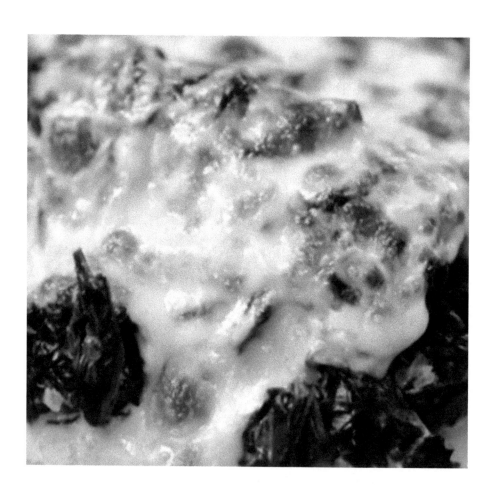

Broccoli, ham, and mozzarella baked with eggs

Ingredients

- 1 teaspoon of spike seasoning
- 10 eggs, beaten well
- 6 cups of chopped broccoli pieces
- 1/3 cup of thinly sliced green onion
- 2 cups of diced ham
- Fresh-ground black pepper
- 1 cup of grated Mozzarella

Directions

- Firstly, heat your oven ready to 375°F.
- Bring a medium-sized pot of water to a boil.
- Cook the broccoli briefly in the boiling water.
- Drain any excess water into a colander.
- Layer broccoli, ham, Mozzarella, and green onions in casserole dish.
- Season with spike seasoning and fresh-ground black pepper.
- Then pour beaten egg over.

- Stir the mixture until all the ingredients are coated with egg.
- Let bake until all the mixture is set in 45 minutes.
- Serve and enjoy with sour cream.

Vegan hummus toasted sandwich

Ingredients

- 3 tablespoons of hummus
- 2 slices of bread
- 1 ripe avocado, thinly sliced
- Salt and pepper
- 1 tablespoon of olive oil
- A handful of rocket
- 4 thin slices of butternut
- ¼ teaspoon of smoked paprika

Directions

- Begin by toasting the slices of bread in a toaster.
- Then, heat 1 tablespoon of the olive oil in a frying pan
- Once hot, add the butternut squash together with the smoked paprika and salt and pepper
- Fry until the squash is soft and golden brown on both sides in 10 minutes or so.
- Spread the hummus on one of the pieces of toasted bread, top with the squash, slices of

avocado, and handful of rocket, combine together.

- Serve and enjoy with lemon squeezed over the avocado.

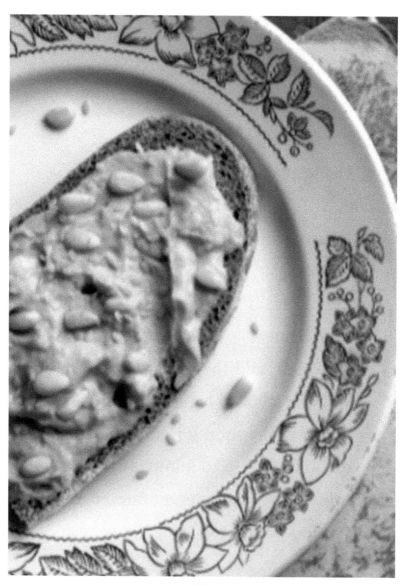

Honey almond ricotta spread with fruit

Ingredients

- Hearty whole grain toast
- Sliced peaches
- 1 cup of whole milk ricotta
- ½ cup of almonds
- ¼ teaspoon of almond extract
- Zest from an orange
- Extra fisher sliced almonds
- 1 teaspoons of honey

Directions

- Combine ricotta together with the almonds and almond extract in a medium sized mixing bowl, stir to combine.
- Transfer to a serving bowl and sprinkle with additional sliced almonds.
- Drizzle with a teaspoon of honey.
- Toast, and spread 1 tablespoon of ricotta on each slice of bread.
- Top with sliced peaches, sliced almonds and honey.
- Serve and enjoy.

Baked eggs with avocado and feta

Ingredients

- Salt and fresh-ground black pepper
- 2 teaspoons of crumbled Feta Cheese
- 1 avocado
- 4 eggs
- Olive oil

Directions

- Break eggs into individual ramekins and let the eggs and avocado come to room temperature.
- Set your oven ready to 400°F.
- Place the gratin dishes on a baking sheet and heat them in the oven for 10 minutes.
- Remove gratin dishes from the oven and spray with olive oil.
- Arrange the sliced avocados in each dish, then, break 2 eggs into each dish.
- Sprinkle with crumbled Feta.
- Then, season with salt and fresh-ground black pepper.

- Let bake until the whites are set and the egg yolks are done to your choice.
- Serve and enjoy.

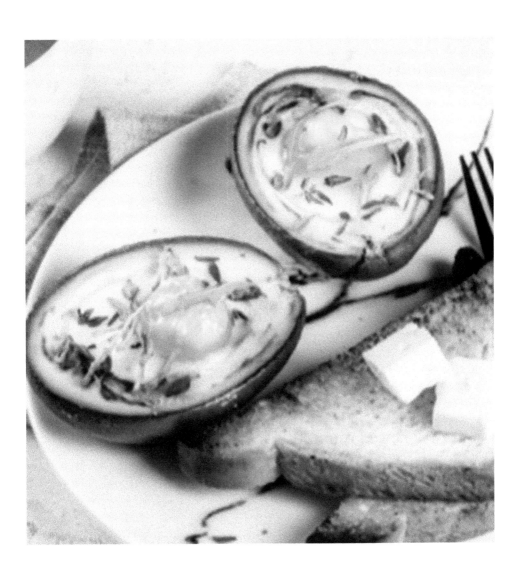

Mediterranean sheet pan salmon

The Mediterranean sheet pan salmon recipe is inspired by Mediterranean ingredients packed with omega 3s. additionally, it features variety of great vegetables for a perfect healthy meal.

Ingredients

- kosher salt and fresh cracked pepper
- 2 small lemons thinly sliced
- ½ cup pitted assorted olives
- Fresh herbs
- 2 tablespoon of salted butter cut in small chunks
- Large whole salmon filet
- 2 cups cherry tomatoes halved
- A few marinated sweet or hot peppers
- 2 teaspoons of capers
- ¼ red onion thinly sliced, rings separated
- 4 tablespoon of extra virgin olive oil

Directions

- Start by preheating your oven ready to 425°F.

- Line a baking sheet with parchment paper and lay out your fish.
- Organize the lemon slices on and around the fish, along with the olives, tomatoes, peppers, capers, and onions.
- Drizzle olive oil all over.
- Sprinkle with salt and pepper.
- Dot with chunks of butter.
- Let bake for 30 minutes, or until the fish is done through.
- Lastly, garnish with fresh herbs.
- Serve and enjoy.

Creamy tomato and roasted veggie risotto

Ingredients

- A small bunch of fresh basil, torn
- Salt and pepper, to taste
- 300g of cherry tomatoes
- 2 red peppers
- 1 large courgette, zucchini
- A generous pinch of salt and pepper
- Vegan parmesan
- 1 tablespoon of olive oil
- 1 large red onion, diced
- 3 garlic cloves, minced
- 1 tablespoon of olive oil
- 225g of risotto rice
- 1 tablespoon of balsamic vinegar
- 250ml of passata
- 250ml of vegetable stock
- 6 sun-dried tomatoes

Directions

- Preheat the oven to 350°F.
- Add the olive oil to a roasting tin.

- Chop and spread vegetables out in the tin.
- Add salt and pepper, shake to coat.
- Let roast for 30 minutes.
- Add olive oil to a shallow casserole dish over a low-medium heat.
- Sauté the onion briefly, then add the minced garlic, cook further for another minute.
- Stir in the rice with the vinegar, stir to coat with the olive oil.
- Pour in the passata and vegetable stock, ½ cup at a time, alternating between the two.
- Let each amount be absorbed by the rice before adding the next.
- After 20 minutes, add in the sundried tomatoes together with the roasted vegetables.
- Remove from the heat and stir in the basil, salt and pepper and vegan cheese.
- Serve and enjoy immediately.

Yogurt tahini Mediterranean carrot salad

Ingredients

- 1/3 cup of crumbled feta
- 2 tablespoons of tahini
- ½ cup of chopped parsley
- 2 tablespoons of water
- Salt and pepper to taste
- ¼ cup of plain Greek yogurt
- 1 tablespoon of lime juice
- ½ tablespoon of honey
- Black sesame seeds for garnish
- 2 large carrots
- 15 ounces can of chickpeas, drained and rinse
- ½ cup of royal raisins

Directions

- Place tahini in a food processor with bit of water. Process until smooth.
- Add the yogurt together with lime juice and honey, process again until smooth.

- Using a spiralizer on blade or a julienne peeler make noodles from the carrots and trim into manageable sizes.
- Place the carrot noodles in a large bowl.
- Add the chickpeas together with the raisins, parsley and feta.
- Add the dressing and toss until well combined.
- Season with salt and pepper to taste.
- Garnish with black sesame seeds.
- Serve and enjoy.

Greek style lemon roasted potatoes

Ingredients

- 1 tablespoon of dried oregano
- 5 lb. Bag of potatoes peeled and quartered
- ¼ cup of olive oil
- 1 lemon juiced
- 1 tablespoon of garlic powder
- 2 teaspoon of salt
- 1 teaspoon of freshly ground pepper

Directions

- Firstly, preheat your oven ready to 400°F.
- Spray a dish with cooking spray and set aside.
- Spread quartered potatoes into an even layer in the pan.
- Juice 1 lemon and pour over the potatoes.
- Cut the lemon peel into small chunks and also add to the pan.
- Add olive oil together with the salt and pepper, oregano, and garlic powder to the pan.
- Stir with a large spoon to combine.

- Let bake for 45 minutes, turning twice with a metal spatula.
- Taste a bite and adjust the seasoning.
- Garnish with parsley, serve and enjoy.

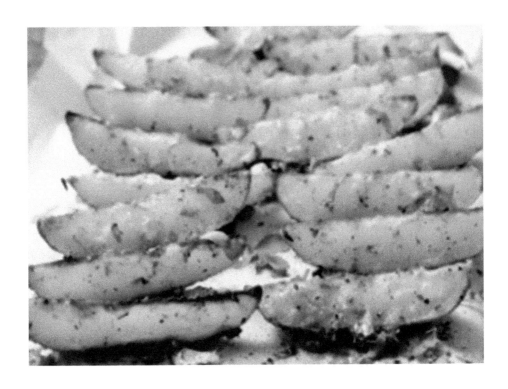

Honey lemon ricotta breakfast toast with figs and pistachios

Ingredients

- 2 tablespoons of pistachio pieces
- 2 slices of whole grain
- 4 figs, sliced
- ¼ cup of low fat ricotta
- 1 teaspoon of lemon zest
- ½ fresh lemon, juiced
- ½ tablespoon of honey

Directions

- Toast bread in toaster.
- Then, whip ricotta together with the lemon juice and honey until smooth and creamy.
- Spread ricotta moisture evenly over each piece of toast.
- Top with sliced figs.
- Sprinkle each piece with pistachio pieces and lemon zest.
- Serve and enjoy.

Breakfast tabbouleh

Ingredients

- ½ cup of bulgur
- 4 tablespoons of olive oil
- 8 large eggs
- 2 cups of fresh Italian flat-leaf parsley, chopped
- ½ pint of grape or cherry tomatoes, diced
- 8 pita wedges
- 1 tablespoon of white vinegar
- ½ cucumber, diced
- Zest and juice of ½ medium lemon
- 1 teaspoon of coarse salt
- ½ teaspoon of ground black pepper

Directions

- Bring 1 cup of water to a boil.
- Then, add bulgur, let cook at a simmer rate for 12 minutes or until water has absorbed, stirring regularly.
- Let cool briefly, then place in an airtight container in the refrigerator until completely cooled.

- In a medium mixing bowl, stir together cooled bulgur, cucumber, lemon juice, olive oil, parsley, tomatoes, salt and pepper.
- Taste, and adjust seasoning accordingly. Place in the refrigerator.
- Bring a large pot of salted water to a simmer.
- Add vinegar and stir to combine.
- Break eggs into the simmering water, one at a time.
- Carefully scoop each egg with a slotted spoon.
- Let eggs cook 3 minutes, until white is set.
- Remove and lay the eggs on a paper towel to dry.
- Scoop tabbouleh and poached eggs on plates.
- Serve and enjoy with pita wedges.

Scrambled eggs in a caramelized onions and paprika

Ingredients

- 2 teaspoons of mixed herb
- 3 tablespoons of Parsley
- 4 Eggs
- 2 tablespoons of olive oil
- 1 medium onion, sliced
- Salt to taste
- 2 teaspoons of chili garlic oil
- 1 large diced tomato
- 1 tablespoon of Feta cheese
- 1 small cube of capsicum
- 3 cloves of garlic, minced
- 2 teaspoons of smoked paprika
- ½ tablespoon of Turmeric

Directions

- Begin by heating the olive oil over medium heat and caramelize onion till they turn dark in 15 minutes.

- Place in the capsicum together with the chili garlic oil. Mix well.
- Add the tomatoes together with the turmeric, garlic, and the mixed herbs.
- Let cook with a tablespoon of water for 5 minutes or so.
- Then, add the paprika.
- Whisk the eggs till frothy.
- Add the eggs, leave to set in 30 seconds.
- Then gently mix it all together.
- Add salt and adjust accordingly to your taste.
- Remove from heat once eggs are set well.
- Lastly, garnish with parsley and feta.
- Serve and enjoy.

Spicy sweet potato hummus

Ingredients

- 1 ½ teaspoon of cayenne pepper
- 2 medium sweet potatoes
- ½ teaspoon of smoked paprika
- 3 tablespoons of olive oil
- ¼ teaspoon of cumin
- 2 cups of cooked chickpeas
- 3 cloves garlic, peeled
- 3 tablespoons of tahini
- zest of ½ lemon
- Ground sea salt, to taste
- juice of 1 lemon

Directions

- Preheat oven to 400°F.
- Bake the sweet potatoes on the middle oven rack for more than 45 minutes.
- Toss all of the other ingredients into a food processor as the potatoes are cooling.
- Add the sweet potatoes to the food processor once the skin is peeled.

- Blend well.
- Serve and enjoy with a light sprinkle of cayenne pepper and sesame seeds.

Vegetarian black bean and sweet potato enchilada

The potatoes are smothered in a salsa Verde with a delicious vegetarian entrée. It features various vegetables for a better taste and flavor.

Ingredients

- 4 ounces of grated cheese
- 1 ¼ pounds sweet potatoes
- 1 can of black beans, rinsed and drained
- 2 tablespoons sour cream
- ¼ cup chopped red onion
- 2 ounces of crumbled feta cheese
- 2 small cans of diced green chilies
- 1 medium jalapeño, seeded and minced
- 2 cloves garlic, pressed or minced
- 1 tablespoon water
- 2 tablespoons lime juice
- ¼ cup chopped fresh cilantro
- ½ teaspoon ground cumin
- ½ teaspoon chili powder
- ¼ teaspoon cayenne pepper

- ¼ teaspoon salt, more to taste
- Freshly ground black pepper
- 2 cups of mild salsa Verde
- 10 corn tortillas

Directions

- Preheat your oven ready to 400°F.
- Line a large baking sheet with parchment paper.
- Place the coated sweet potatoes with oil, flat-side down on the baking sheet.
- Bake for 35 minutes or until tender and cooked through.
- Pour enough salsa Verde into a baking dish to lightly cover the bottom
- In a medium mixing bowl, combine cumin, lime juice, cayenne pepper, chili powder, garlic, jalapeno, green chilies, feta cheese, jack cheese, beans, salt, and ground black pepper.
- Scoop out the potato flesh with a spoon. Lightly mash them with a fork.
- Stir the mashed sweet potato into the bowl of filling, and season to taste.

- Warm up your tortillas, in a skillet, wrap them in a clean tea towel to maintain the warmth.
- Working with one tortilla at a time, spread about ½ cup filling down the center each tortilla, then wrap both sides over the filling and place it in the baking dish.
- Repeat for all of the tortillas.
- Top with the remaining salsa Verde and cheese.
- Bake for 35 minutes, until sauce is bubbling.
- Let cool and drizzle with sour cream.
- Serve and enjoy.

Roasted vegetable enchilada casserole

Unlike other Mediterranean Sea diet recipes, this one takes a different turn of featuring hearty fresh Mexican vegetable flavors. It a main dish and gluten free.

Ingredients

- ½ cup of chopped fresh cilantro
- 10 corn tortillas, halved
- ½ medium head of cauliflower, cut into chunks
- 1 large sweet potato, peeled and cut into cubes
- Freshly ground black pepper
- 1 can of black beans, rinsed and drained
- 2 red bell peppers, cut into 1" squares
- 2 cups shredded Jack cheese
- 1 medium yellow onion, sliced into wedges
- 3 tablespoons of extra-virgin olive oil, divided
- 2 big handfuls of baby spinach leaves
- 1 teaspoon of ground cumin, divided
- Salt
- 2 ¼ cups of red salsa

Directions

- Preheat your oven ready to 400°F.
- Line 2 large, baking sheets with parchment paper.
- Combine the cauliflower and sweet potato in one pan.
- On the other, combine the bell peppers together with the onion.
- Drizzle half of the olive oil over one pan, and the other half over the other pan.
- Sprinkle them lightly with salt and pepper, toss to coat vegetables in oil and spices.
- Arrange the vegetables in an even layer across each pan.
- Let bake until the vegetables are tender on the edges, for 35 minutes, tossing and swapping the pans halfway.
- Lower the oven heat and lightly grease square baker. Then, stir the cilantro into the salsa.
- Spread ½ cup salsa evenly over the bottom of the baking pan.
- Add a single layer of halved tortilla pieces.

- Top with beans, vegetables, spinach, and ⅓ of the cheese.
- Make a second layer of tortillas topping with remaining components.
- Make many layers as you can.
- Cover the pan with parchment paper, let bake for 20 minutes, then remove the parchment paper, let bake for 10 more minutes.
- Serve and enjoy.

Mason jar chickpea, faro, and greens salad

Ingredients

- Handful of dried cherries
- 1 ¼ cup of faro
- ¼ cup of pepitas
- 1 tablespoon of olive oil
- 1 medium clove garlic, pressed or minced
- Kalamata olives, pitted and thinly sliced
- ¼ teaspoon salt
- ½ cup of red wine vinegar
- 4 cloves garlic, pressed or minced
- 4 stalks celery, thinly sliced and roughly chopped
- Feta cheese, crumbled
- 1 tablespoon of dried oregano
- 2 teaspoons of Dijon mustard
- ⅓ cup of Greek dressing
- 1 teaspoon of freshly ground black pepper
- 1 teaspoon of agave nectar, honey or sugar
- 2 cans of chickpeas, drained and rinsed

- ⅔ cup of chopped red onion
- 1 cup of chopped parsley
- Mixed greens

Directions

- In a medium saucepan, combine the rinsed faro together with 3 cups water
- Bring the water to a boil, then reduce heat to a gentle simmer, until the faro is tender.
- Drain any excess water and mix in the olive oil together with the garlic and salt. Let cool.
- Then, whisk together extra virgin olive oil, red wine vinegar, garlic, dried oregano, Dijon mustard, salt, ground black pepper, and agave nectar until emulsified.
- In a serving bowl, toss together the chickpeas together with the prepared celery, red onion, and parsley. Stir in enough dressing to coat the salad. Toss and set aside.
- In another skillet over medium heat, toast the pepitas for a few minutes, stirring frequently, until they smell toasty.
- Let cool in a bowl.

- In a quart-sized mason jar, layer the chickpea salad at the bottom with an additional tablespoon of dressing.
- Top with cooled faro and greens.
- Serve and enjoy.

Feta fiesta kale salad with avocado and crispy tortilla strips

This recipe combines broad ingredients ranging from vegetables and fruit juice with herbs. Therefore, it is a perfect choice of Mediterranean Sea diet.

Ingredients

- In a small bowl, whisk olive oil together with lime juice, jalapeno, honey, ground honey, coriander, and pinch of salt until emulsified.
- Place chopped and sliced kale to a big salad bowl.
- Sprinkle with a small pinch of sea salt, then massage the leaves with hands at a time, until the leaves turn darker and fragrant.
- Drizzle salad dressing over the kale and toss well t coat.
- Add the drained black beans together with the feta, avocado and chopped cilantro to mixing bowl.
- In a skillet over medium-low heat toast the pepitas for briefly, stirring frequently, until fragrant.

- Transfer to the salad bowl. Toss to combine.
- Stack the corn tortillas and slice them into thin little strips.
- Heat a large pan drizzled with olive oil over medium heat.
- Toss in the tortilla slices when the olive oil begins to shimmer, sprinkle with salt and stir.
- Let cook until the strips are crispy and turning golden in 5 minutes, stirring occasionally.
- Remove tortilla strips from skillet and drain on a plate covered with a piece of paper towel.
- Serve and enjoy topped with salad and crispy tortilla strips.

Thai mango cabbage wraps with crispy tofu and peanut sauce

The Thai mango cabbage wrap is a wonderfully delicious Mediterranean Sea diet recipe with healthy peanut sauce, cabbage as a salad wrap is irresistible.

Ingredients

- ⅓ cup of packed fresh cilantro leaves, chopped
- 1 block of organic extra-firm tofu
- 1 medium red bell pepper, chopped
- 1 jalapeño, minced
- 1 tablespoon of olive oil
- 2 garlic cloves, pressed
- ¼ teaspoon salt
- 1 tablespoon of reduced-sodium tamari
- 2 teaspoons of arrowroot
- 2 tablespoons large, <u>unsweetened coconut flakes</u>
- ⅓ cup of creamy peanut butter
- 2 tablespoons of white wine vinegar
- 2 tablespoons chopped peanuts
- 1 small head of green cabbage

- 2 tablespoons of honey
- 2 teaspoons of toasted sesame oil
- 1 lime, juiced
- 2 ripe mangos, diced
- ½ bunch of green onions, chopped

Directions

- Preheat your oven ready to 400°F.
- Drain the tofu completely.
- Slice tofu into thirds.
- Transfer to a plate lined with paper towels.
- Fold the towel over one tofu slab, then place the other slab on top.
- Repeat with the last slab.
- Whisk together peanut butter, white wine vinegar, tamari, honey, sesame oil, and garlic until well blended.
- Transfer the drained tofu to a cutting board.
- Slice each slab into four columns and four rows.
- Whisk together 1 tablespoon olive oil and tamari, then drizzle it over the tofu and toss to coat.

- Sprinkle 1 teaspoon arrowroot starch over the tofu, toss to incorporated.
- Let bake for 35 minutes, tossing, until the tofu is deeply golden.
- Combine mangos, red bell pepper, green onions, cilantro leaves, jalapeno, lime juice, and salt in a small serving bowl, toss.
- Pull off one leaf at a time. Repeat until you have 8 cabbage leaves.
- Toast the coconut flakes and chopped peanuts over medium heat, stirring frequently, until the coconut is golden.
- Add the tofu to the pan. Pour in the peanut sauce, toss to coat. Cook, until the tofu has absorbed the sauce.
- Serve and enjoy.

Strawberry kale salad with nutty granola croutons

A combination of raw vegetables and fruits mainly red kale, strawberries, radishes with crumbled cheese is healthy for any individual.

Ingredients

- ½ cup of raw sunflower seeds
- 8 ounces of kale
- ½ cup of whole almonds
- ¼ cup of raw sesame seeds
- ½ pound of strawberries, hulled and sliced
- 5 medium radishes, sliced thin and roughly chopped
- 1 tablespoon of fennel seeds
- 2 ounces of chilled goat cheese
- 1 cup of old-fashioned oats
- ¼ teaspoon of cayenne pepper
- 3 tablespoons of olive oil
- 2 tablespoons of lemon juice
- 1 tablespoon of smooth Dijon mustard
- 1 large egg white, beaten

- 2 ½ teaspoons of honey
- Sea salt and freshly ground pepper, to taste
- ½ cup of raw shelled pistachios

Directions

- Preheat oven to 350°F.
- Then, in a medium bowl, toss oats together with the sunflower seeds, sesame seeds, fennel seeds, pistachios, almonds, salt, and cayenne pepper.
- Stir in the beaten egg white with olive oil, and honey, until blended.
- Transfer mixture to baking sheet.
- Let bake, stirring halfway, until golden in 19 minutes. Allow it to cool on the baking sheet.
- In another small mixing bowl, whisk together the olive oil with lemon juice, mustard, and honey until emulsified.
- Season with sea salt and freshly ground black pepper.
- Transfer the chopped kale to a big salad bowl.
- Sprinkle with a small pinch of sea salt and massage the leaves with your hands.

- Drizzle in the salad dressing, toss well, until all of the kale is lightly coated in dressing.
- Add the sliced strawberries and chopped radishes, then use a fork to crumble the goat cheese over the salad.
- Serve and enjoy.

Sugar snap pea and carrot soba noodles

The sugar snap pea and carrot soba noodles recipe features a highly vibrant fresh springtime produce good enough for a Mediterranean Sea diet.

Ingredients

- 1 tablespoon of white miso
- 6 ounces of soba noodles
- 2 cups of frozen organic edamame
- 10 ounces of sugar snap peas
- 1 tablespoon of toasted sesame oil
- 6 medium-sized carrots, peeled
- 1 tablespoon of honey
- 1 teaspoon of chili garlic sauce
- ½ cup of chopped fresh cilantro
- 1 small lime, juiced
- ¼ cup of sesame seeds
- 2 teaspoons of freshly grated ginger
- ¼ cup of reduced-sodium tamari
- 2 tablespoons of peanut oil

Directions

- Whisk together tamari, peanut oil, lemon juice, sesame oil, honey, white miso, ginger, and chili garlic sauce in a small bowl until emulsified. Keep aside for later.
- Bring 2 big pots of water to a boil.
- As the water boils, pour the sesame seeds into a small pan. Toast for 5 minutes over medium heat, shaking the pan frequently, until the seeds are turning golden.
- Cook the soba noodles according to package Directions in the boiling water.
- Drain any excess water and rinse under cool water.
- Then, cook the frozen edamame in the other pot until warmed through in 6 minutes.
- Toss the halved peas into the boiling edamame water and cook for an additional 20 seconds. Drain.
- Combine the soba noodles together with the edamame, snap peas, and carrots in a large serving bowl.

- Pour in the dressing, toss with salad servers.
- Serve and enjoy tossed in the chopped cilantro and toasted sesame seeds. Serve.

Lemony lentil and chickpea salad with radish and herbs

This recipe blends beans with lemon and mint flavor. It takes only 20 minutes for the chickpea and lentils to get ready for your lunch or dinner.

Ingredients

- 2 cups of dried black beluga lentils
- 1 big bunch of radishes, sliced thin and roughly chopped
- Freshly ground black pepper, to taste
- 2 large garlic cloves, halved lengthwise
- ¼ cup of chopped fresh, leafy herbs, chopped
- 1 clove of garlic, pressed or minced
- 4 tablespoons of olive oil
- 1 can of chickpeas, rinsed and drained
- ¼ cup of fresh lemon juice
- Sliced avocado, crumbled feta
- 1 teaspoon of Dijon mustard
- 1 teaspoon of honey
- ¼ teaspoon of fine-grain sea salt

Directions

- In a medium pot, combine the lentils together with garlic cloves, olive oil and 4 cups water.
- Bring the water to a boil, then lower the heat, let simmer and cook until the lentils tender in 35 minutes max.
- Drain the lentils and discard the garlic cloves.
- Whisk together the chickpeas, radishes, fresh herbs, and avocado slices in a small bowl.
- In a large serving bowl, combine the lentils together with the chickpeas, chopped radishes and herbs.
- Drizzle in the dressing and toss to combine.
- Serve and enjoy with avocado, crumbled cheese and or fresh greens.

Roasted cherry tomato, arugula and sorghum salad

The presence of sorghum makes this recipe quite unique and truly Mediterranean with other various vegetables with a lemon dressing. It is quite healthy; the sorghum is a greater source of carbohydrates as the chickpea is a greater source of proteins.

Ingredients

- 3 cups of baby arugula
- 1 cup of sorghum, rinsed
- ¼ cup of crumbled feta
- 3 cups of water
- 1 can of chickpeas, rinsed and drained
- ¼ teaspoon of fine grain sea salt
- 1 pint of cherry tomatoes
- Sea salt
- 3 tablespoons olive oil
- 2 tablespoons of lemon juice
- 2 tablespoons of grated Parmesan cheese
- ¼ teaspoon of red pepper flakes
- 1 clove of garlic, pressed

- Freshly ground black pepper, to taste

Directions

- Combine rinsed sorghum with water in a small pot.
- Bring to a boil, covered, then lower the heat to medium-low.
- Cook until the sorghum is pleasantly tender In 66 minutes.
- Then, preheat your oven to 400°F.
- Line a small, baking sheet with parchment paper.
- Toss the whole cherry tomatoes with 1 tablespoon of olive oil, then sprinkle with salt.
- Let, roast for 18 minutes, or until the tomatoes are plump and starting to burst open.
- Whisk together the red pepper flakes, olive oil, lemon juice, salt and pepper until emulsified.
- Drain off any excess water out of the sorghum, pour into a serving bowl.
- Pour in all of the dressing, all of the cherry tomatoes and their juices, the arugula, feta,

Parmesan and chickpeas, then, give it a big toss.

- Serve and enjoy.

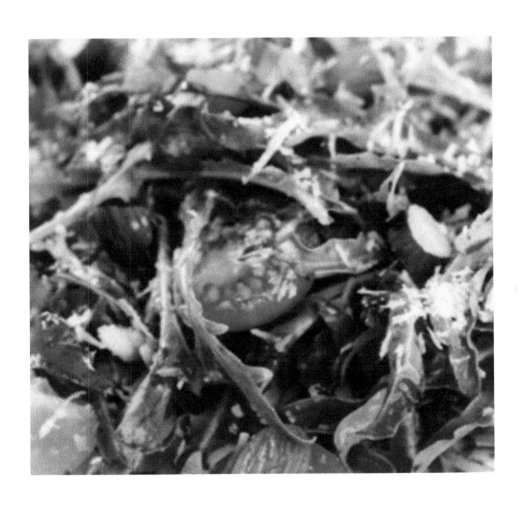

Spring carrot, radish, and quinoa salad with herbed avocado

In a simple lemon vinaigrette, this recipe features several vegetables such as carrots, fennel, garlicky, radishes, quinoa, and herbed avocado for a perfect Mediterranean Sea diet choice.

Ingredients

- 2 garlic cloves, pressed or minced
- 1 small lime or lemon, juiced
- 2 ½ teaspoons of olive oil
- 3 packed tablespoons of fresh herbs
- 4 cups of arugula
- ⅛ teaspoon of sea salt
- 2 radishes, sliced into strips
- Lots of freshly ground black pepper
- 3 carrots, peeled and then sliced into ribbons
- ¼ bulb fennel, cored and sliced thinly
- 3 tablespoons of sunflower seeds
- 3 tablespoons of crumbled feta
- 1 lemon, zested and juiced
- Dash sea salt

- ½ cup of quinoa, rinsed
- ½ teaspoon o ground coriander
- 1 teaspoon of Dijon mustard
- ½ teaspoon honey or agave nectar
- 1 large avocado, diced

Directions

- In a saucepan, combine the quinoa and 1 cup water.
- Bring the mixture to a boil, covered, then lower the heat to a simmer.
- Let cook for 15 minutes, remove let it rest, for 5 minutes.
- Fluff the quinoa and mix in the garlic with the olive oil.
- Season, and adjust accordingly.
- Pour the seeds into a small pan.
- Heat the seeds over medium heat, stirring frequently, until turning golden on the edges. Remove.
- In a small bowl, whisk the olive oil together with the lemon juice and zest, mustard, and honey until emulsified.

- Season with sea salt and black pepper.
- In another separate small bowl, combine the chunks of avocado, chopped fresh herbs, lemon or lime juice, coriander, and sea salt.
- Mash with a fork until the mixture is blended.
- Divide the arugula and quinoa between two large salad bowls.
- Then, drizzle with vinaigrette lightly, and toss to coat.
- Divide the radishes, carrots, and fennel between the two bowls.
- Top with a sprinkling of sunflower seeds and feta cheese.
- Serve and enjoy.